WELLNESS JOURNEYS

America's Top Professionals Share Stories of

Real People Overcoming Real Health Issues

Without Drugs or Surgery

Volume One

Wellness Journeys :
America's Top Professionals Share Stories of
Real People Overcoming Real Health Issues
Without Drugs or Surgery

Copyright © 2015 by C. Anthony Curtis

Readers, for more information,
visit facebook.com/wellnessjourneys2015

Wellness Professionals, for more information,
visit rpmpublish.com

Book and Cover design by RPM Publishing

Cover Image Credit: aarmono @ flickr.com

ISBN: 0692459588

CONTENTS

INTRODUCTION

" The first wealth is health."

~ Ralph Waldo Emerson

There is no denying the value of good health. When you feel good, life is good. When you don't, it isn't. Yet many of us don't invest much time or energy into maximizing our health.

I'm not just talking about diet and exercise.

Even when something is obviously wrong with our bodies, most people just follow the status quo. They go to their doctor and get one of three answers: 1) drugs, 2) surgery, or 3) nothing can be done about it. I'm not a big fan of any of those answers.

Our bodies were designed to heal themselves, without the intervention of laboratory chemicals or another human being carving us up like a Thanksgiving turkey. And I really can't stand when an opinion like "nothing can be done" is stated as if it were a fact.

Alternative medical treatments have been proven to work for many years now, yet change is difficult for most people. They'd rather stay stuck in a comfortable rut, than take the time to discover for themselves all of the possible solutions available for their health issues.

Clearly, I'm not talking about you because you're reading this book. Congratulations on not being a rut dweller!

I must admit I used to be a rut dweller, until I had my eyes opened by a personal medical situation. My wife, daughter and I were involved in a serious car accident when a truck lost control late one rainy night on the 101 freeway just South of San Francisco.

Our injuries led us to our first experience with the benefits of chiropractic services. The results were amazing! After unsuccessfully trying to manage our pain with drugs, we found our back and neck pain disappeared almost immediately.

If you're living with pain or other health issues, especially those mentioned in this book, you owe it to yourself to learn how others have successfully conquered their ailments with the help of a natural wellness professional.

You will read stories of people who spent their entire lives dealing with the pain of chronic migraines, only to find the solution was simple.

Many people think chiropractic services are only for neck and back pain, but that couldn't be further from the truth. In this book, you'll read stores of relief from migraines, seizures, eczema, high blood pressure, diabetes, arthritis, tremors, fatigue, fainting, incontinence, anxiety, depression, low libido and a few others.

This could have been a simple "how to" book that listed ailments with their corresponding treatments, but where's the fun in that? Plus, you want proven treatments that have produced results for others, right? Unproven theories are a dime a dozen.

We wanted to inspire our readers and give them hope, so we searched high and low for wellness professionals who had successfully treated these ailments. Well, we found them -- and they have been amazing partners in the production of this book.

They have agreed to provide full contact information so readers who have questions about their treatment plans can contact them directly!

I guarantee that by the time you get to the last page of this book, you will have a whole new perspective on modern medical solutions.

This book could be the first step in your journey towards a full recovery from your own condition and better health overall.

~ Anthony Curtis

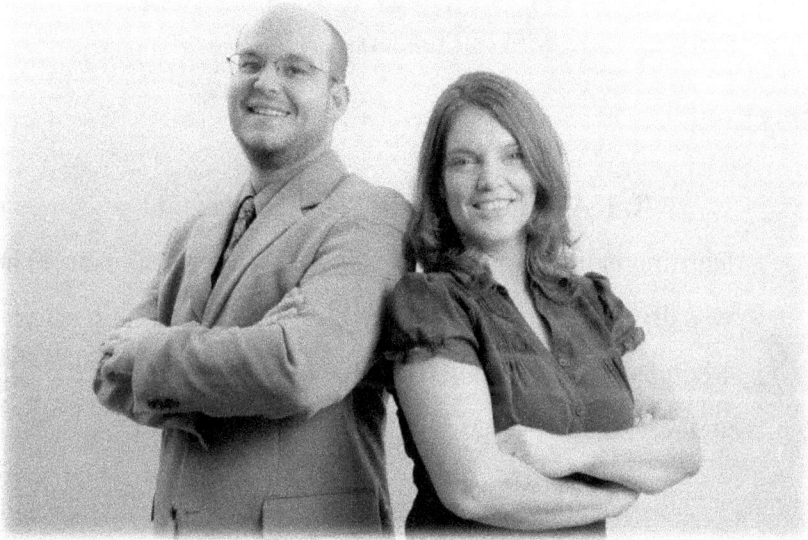

Drs. Katy & Ted Morter, IV

*Share Inspiring Stories of Relief from
Headaches, Stomach Pain, Emotional Stress,
Seizures, Speech Impediments and Eczema*

ANTHONY: Dr. Katy, welcome to the Wellness Journeys interview series. I know you have an exciting personal wellness story to share with our readers.

DR. KATY MORTER: The excitement that comes from learning is infectious and I believe my interest in natural health was driven from watching my father in Osteopathic school when I was very young – between the formative ages of three and six.

Osteopathy changed, however, and by the time I was in college, all I heard from my family was "don't go into medicine." They complained about drug companies, regulation and malpractice rates and were, quite simply, miserable. They didn't practice Osteopathy anymore. They practiced medicine – just like most M.D.s – a pill or surgery for every woe. So, I listened to them, and changed my degree focus from Pre-Med. After years of a wide variety of desk jobs (and careers – I just couldn't seem to find my passion!), headaches crippled my life.

I was working as a web graphics artist, sitting slouched in front of a computer in a stressful job, in a stressful marriage, in the stressful Washington, DC suburbs. I was miserable! It was a recipe for health disaster. I understood enough to be dangerous about natural health. My diet was fairly good - not great, I didn't take medications and was on the "this is the next greatest supplement" bandwagon.

Finally, my body had enough of my poor posture and even poorer attitude. A headache developed at the base of my skull that wouldn't go away with yoga, my wonderful massage therapist, or any of the gadgets I'd bought to help "alleviate neck tension and realign the vertebrae."

When I thought it couldn't get any worse, a co-worker sidled up to my cubicle to tell me how wonderful he felt. He had just come back from his Chiropractor. I didn't know anything about Chiropractic – except that it was like Osteopathy. I was in pain and my co-worker had his Chiropractor's card right there, so I made an appointment with Dr. Nick Triandos. Then, my appointment was postponed. He had a "Chiropractic emergency!" I'd never heard of such a thing and thought it was an excuse. It turns out, a patient had injured herself pretty badly and couldn't leave her house that was about an hour away. So, Dr. Triandos went to her.

I've since had to rearrange my schedule due to "Chiropractic emergencies" several times, and my patients are always very understanding.

When I finally did meet Dr. Triandos the next day, I felt very comfortable with him - very unlike other doctors' visits I'd had in the past. After an explanation of the nervous system and an exam, I had my first adjustment -- Cracks, pops and twists on my neck and back! It scared me senseless! But, immediately felt my headache fade! On my way back to my office that lunchtime, I decided I wanted to be a Chiropractor.

After a couple of years of finishing up some college requirements and saving up some money, I moved to Dallas, Texas to begin Chiropractic school. My husband didn't go with me.

It was during my first semester at school, I met two people who would completely change my perspective, my life and my wellness journey.

The first was a young Chiropractor who had just begun teaching in the clinic. In fact, it was my fortune to encounter him on his first day. No one else was around except me, my befuddled intern and this guy. My headaches continued – I needed to get adjusted regularly to keep them at bay – and my poor intern just couldn't make a dent in them. Frustrated, she asked the young man watching us "She keeps complaining about headaches! What should I do?"

He calmly said, "Adjust her atlas." The atlas is the top vertebrae in the spine and – I've since learned – a hotbed area of nervous system cell bodies that control the entire body.

My intern had no idea on how to adjust an atlas. (Most Atlas Chiropractors, me included, take several hours of post-graduate classes to become masters of their trade.) So, it was here I received my very first Upper Cervical adjustment from Dr. Paul Collett. No cracking, popping or twisting which I still didn't particularly care for – just a gentle drop on a short table.

I immediately felt a rush of heat to my face and my neck felt better. I still had a little headache but, honestly, I didn't think it would ever completely go away. In fact, I had – along with most people – resigned myself to the "fact" that I would have a little bit of pain forever. I thought people who said they felt fantastic were lying. As I was getting older, there would always be some sort of pain.

But I would be proven wrong! Two weeks and a couple more adjustments later, my neck tension and headaches had decreased substantially. Then, it happened. I was sitting at a stoplight and realized I had no discomfort in my body! I felt FANTASTIC!

I was hooked, and wanted to learn as much as I could about how to adjust "the atlas."

My wellness journey, however, was far from finished.

As I mentioned, my life had been pretty stressful before school. In fact, it had been pretty stressful my whole life – but that's a much longer story. School was an eye opener! I only had myself to worry about and I was able to focus on my studies and my body. And what I learned from listening to my body was that when I was more stressed, my adjustments didn't hold as well, my stomach hurt and that headache would creep back in like the pain-in-the-neck that it truly was.

That's when I met Ted Morter, IV.

Ted was a classmate who I had only met briefly for the first couple months in school. His grandfather had been president of the college and most teachers knew who he was. I had no idea.

One day, after an extremely fascinating anatomy lecture – at least, to me it was fascinating - a group of us were talking about the circulatory system in the digestive tract. BEAUTIFUL! It was soon obvious that only one other person was as stoked as I was – and that was Ted. Everyone else left.

Our fondness and excitement about the body led to me asking him why everyone knew his grandfather. It turned out to be the missing piece of the puzzle that I had been searching for – in more ways than I could imagine.

Whereas most of the chiropractic techniques I had been associated with were purely structural, Ted's grandfather, whose name was also Ted, had created a technique that addressed the emotional aspects of why people's bodies become imbalanced and go out of alignment.

The technique, Bio-Energetic Synchronization Technique (B.E.S.T. – there were a lot of jokes in school about that), doesn't just address current emotional stress. It looks to the origin of that stress – often what could have started in childhood!

After being treated by Ted and other students who were in the B.E.S.T. club at school, I no longer suffered from the same level of physical tension caused by stressful events like my mother calling.

My soon-to-be-former husband, who I had always walked on eggshells around, didn't create the same dread. I felt physically better and happier than ever before.

My body felt fantastic. My brain felt fantastic. I decided that these two approaches that had helped me would be the central focus of my relationship with my clients.

A couple years later, the friendship that Ted and I fostered developed into something deeper and we began a life together. After five years in practice, these two very different (but very compatible) methods have allowed us to create amazing changes in our clients from across the country.

VOLUME ONE

ANTHONY: Thank you for sharing your personal wellness story, Dr. Katy! Now tell us about that worried mother who came to you for help with her son's seizures.

DR. KATY MORTER: The voice on the other end of the phone sounded like a woman at the edge of sanity. I'd often taken calls from people asking if we could help them in our clinic, with conditions as varied as headaches to cancer, but this woman was THE most desperate I'd encountered.

I listened as Julia talked – for about an hour – about her son, Philip. He was a bright, funny boy about 10 years old who was a straight-A student and the third in a family of six kids.

Julia had been a young mom and was doing her best to raise healthy, smart kids. Her first two had been easy, but over the past year Philip had experienced epileptic seizures lasting about six seconds.

Afraid for the health of her child, Julia put him on the anti-seizure medication recommended by their neurologist.

The medicine didn't work.

Not only didn't it stop or even reduce the seizures, it turned a bright, straight-A boy into a gloomy, angry failing student.

The medical doctor told her to keep him on the medication but to add another one that would temper the psychological effects from the first. Julia said, "No."

This was where I entered the story. The woman on the other end of the phone wasn't just calling to help her son, she was trying to save her family. When she took her son off the medication, the school got involved.

The Department of Human Services threatened to take all of her children away – if she didn't keep her son on a medication that wasn't working!

Her last hope was to quickly create a change in Philip's health and she had heard Chiropractic could possibly help. She was grasping at straws and needed someone to give her a bit of hope. I told her I couldn't promise an end to his seizures, but that we would do everything we could to help them.

I rearranged a few appointments and she drove an hour-and-a-half to bring Philip to see me that afternoon. When I saw Philip, I couldn't believe the look on this boy's face. His poor, tired eyes were ringed with dark circles and he sat slumped in his chair, defeated.

I had already heard Philip's story from his mom, so when I asked him about his seizures, he just said they were "kinda scary." He didn't talk much, so I just explained to him what I tell all my patients: that a part of the brain runs his body without him knowing.

Most of the time, the subconscious brain communicates with every cell in the body to coordinate filtering, cleansing, digesting, and resting. Stress, however, causes the body to change.

When the stress mode takes over, the body goes into defense mode, ready to mobilize all its energy for one goal – to stay alive. Things like digesting food, reproduction, proper filtering of toxins, thinking – they are a waste of energy in that moment.

Increased blood pressure, heart rate, blood sugar and shallow breathing help us get away from – or fight – a threat. Most people experience tension or anxiety. When these things happened to Philip, however, he had a seizure.

Lately, there had been a lot of seizures – and a lot of family stress. Feeling guilty for causing his family such pain, Philip hadn't been sleeping much either, which led to even more seizures. After I told him how the brain runs the body, and how stress could be a big factor in getting rid of his seizures, he looked relieved.

Our clinic is different than most Chiropractic clinics. We have a very simply approach – get the brain and body talking to each other efficiently and they'll do most of the work.

For Philip, we gently adjusted the top bone in his spine that is tethered to the spinal cord. Then we worked on how his body is responding to his thoughts and emotions (and there were a lot of emotions tied up in this little guy!) with a Bio-Energetic Synchronization Technique treatment.

They came back the next week with the seizures cut in half the length. From six seconds, they went down to three. Success, but still not good enough. We had to move! That's when we came to the family overhaul.

The "healthy" diet they had been eating was mostly processed food. Breakfast was a frozen biscuit sandwich and, as the mom of six kids, Julia had her hands full just trying to get them to eat anything.

It's funny what an ultimatum will do. The family diet instantly changed. Julia bought organic vegetables when she could and started making fresh meals for not just Philip, but the entire clan.

With the school officials breathing down her neck, we had to do some drastic changes for Philip to see if he had any dietary stress triggers, but he was ready. So, he got rid of the usual suspects – sugar, dairy, gluten, soy.

After a few weeks, he was almost completely seizure free! And we'd even determined that sugar was the main culprit and he was able to include more things back into his diet.

Even the school health official who had spearheaded this whole episode (and put me through the fifth degree on the phone) admitted that Philip was doing great. He couldn't believe it! Everything was going great, that is, until…….
GRANDMA.

You see, Grandma didn't like it that her little grandson wasn't allowed to have sugar. AND, it was someone's birthday. AND, all kids should be able to have a piece of cake. (Julia wasn't at this event, by the way.) So, Philip ate a piece of cake.

Julia had explained the situation to me over the phone when I saw them two days later. Philip – who had been seizure free for several weeks - had not one, but three seizures at school the day after eating the cake. He had been sent home for the day. It was a sobering blow to all of us, especially Julia.

As Philip lay on the table waiting for an adjustment, I began to talk to him – and here's where it got really interesting. I casually said, "So, I heard you had a piece of cake." Upon hearing the word "cake," Philip had a seizure.

Just the thought of cake caused his brain to react in a seizure!

When he had recovered, I treated him on his stressful emotional reaction to the word cake and repeated the exact phrase "So, I heard you had a piece of cake." -- this time, nothing, except a gasp from his mama.

While he was resting after the upper cervical adjustment, Julia and I had a little talk. She was the defender of her kids and felt betrayed by a family member who "knew best" and thought she was "too strict on the kids." I offered to have a little talk with Grandma, but it turns out I didn't have to. She'd figured it out on her own.

There would continue to be a few hiccups now and again, but Philip just kept having fewer and fewer seizures. . Instead of being on medication for a lifetime, without finding the root cause of his seizures, Philip was now eating healthily with a different picture of how his body works.

Now, he's in high school and a wrestler and a brilliant student.

And he wasn't the only one who changed. The entire family is now healthier thanks to Julia's diet and lifestyle overhaul!

ANTHONY: Wow that was another amazing wellness journey, Dr. Katy! Got another one for us?

DR. KATY MORTER: Many times a patient will come to our office with one problem in mind, but discover that there are much more important and critical issues that need to be addressed – issues that will affect not only their lives, but their entire family as well.

Little Clara was scheduled to see me for tongue-tie issues. She was about a year old and was tiny for her age, but very well-fed.

Her mom was a beautiful lady with a gentle British accent, but from the moment she sat down, I could tell she was under a great deal of stress – and that was affecting everything and everybody in her family.

Now stress isn't unusual with moms whose babies aren't eating well. Nothing creates more stress for a mother than a baby who isn't thriving.

I had seen a lot of success with babies with these restrictions and much of that success was due to helping the mother realize how her emotions affect her baby. Mom became less stressed, so the baby healed much more quickly with my and other dental treatments.

But the stress for Emma was deeper. The first thing I noticed was that the side of poor Clara's face was covered with a scab. I thought she'd had an accident and was astounded to hear that it was "just eczema." Immediately, our simple tongue-tie conversation turned deeper.

Clara was the youngest of three children and her father had left them just after she was born – and had another baby about Clara's age, to boot! Talk about stress!

Already riddled with emotional strain, Emma had tried everything to relieve the eczema. She eliminated the typical "suspect" foods from her diet – dairy, gluten, sugar, soy, meat. Nothing had helped.

Creams, oils, herbs – nothing could change that nasty, itchy rash on her face. Poor Clara was miserable and way more anxious than a toddler should be and poor Emma was about ready to crack!

I agreed to take Clara on as a patient and told Emma that the stress level in the family was a going to be a huge factor in Clara's success of both latching better and healing the eczema.

Because their stress was continuous and didn't seem to have a quick solution, I advised Emma that it might take a while to see results.

After the first adjustment, Clara's latch was much improved. Her eczema was less itchy, for a day – then came back full force.

At the next appointment, Emma brought in her beautiful 10-year old daughter, Simone, for an adjustment as well. Just for fun, I put Emma on the table for a quick, gentle balancing of the stress-related part of her nervous system. It was time for Christmas break and I asked Emma to consider treatments for the entire family.

Two weeks passed and the next time I saw Emma and her family at first glance, not much had changed. Emma was still stressed out and little Clara's face was still red and scabby however, Emma was excited to begin family treatments!

I didn't know it, but before coming to see me initially, she had, herself, been seeing a Chiropractor for a jaw injury that happened when she tripped over a dishwasher door – while in an argument with her former husband.

The emotional charge surrounding the injury kept her body from being able to heal. Unbeknownst to me, we addressed that issue during her brief treatment before Christmas and the debilitating pain vanished!

The entire family began to get regular gentle treatments of their vertebrae and other joints as well as the mind-body methods we use to treat emotional restrictions.

As much as I wanted to help this family heal, the stress of their daily lives made it impossible to create a lasting change with only adjustments. They needed their own tools to help them reduce their stress at home.

So, we started with the most basic and simple, but most amazingly effective stress-buster of them all: Breathing.

First, I had Emma set an alarm on her phone every hour to remind her to take a few deep breaths -- nothing specific, just deep breaths.

Make things too complicated and people won't do them, especially moms, who homeschool, and are nannies, like Emma....

So, she began her "breathe breaks." She began to feel less stressed at home. The kids began to be less stressed, and there was less for me to do when they came in for their adjustments. Little Clara's face, however, was improved, but not as much as I'd hoped.

Now it was time to experiment. I asked Emma to hold Clara during her breathe breaks, to let Clara feel her mother's body relaxing.

I wondered if that could be a catalyst to help turn this on-guard, anxious little girl into the giggly squigglebox of which we'd rarely caught a glimpse.

One week later, on their next visit, the change was remarkable! The redness on her face was almost completely gone!

The stress from her father was still looming, but her body wasn't reacting to it so severely!

Emma was overjoyed! I was ecstatic! And little Clara was smiling! It was a jaw-dropping moment as a doctor and I was overcome with the beauty of this little body's healing powers!

As the weeks went on, the healing continued. When Emma became too stressed, Clara's face would break out and Emma would double her efforts to stay calm.

If her father created drama in their lives, Clara's face would break out – but never as brutally as before. Clara's face became a barometer of just how much they let stress get to them.

Lastly, Emma was able to add foods back into their diet with no adverse reaction. They still eat healthily, just with more options.

Now, the three kids know when they need an adjustment. Simone, the sassy ten-year old, will tell her mother when she feels angry but can't explain it and needs to be treated.

Little Clara will stop and breathe when she can't get to something she wants, or her brother and sister lock her out of a room.

The most exciting part, for me as their doctor, is seeing this mother take charge of her beautiful family.

She was feeling more confident and relaxed when thinking about their future and seeing children become aware of their bodies and the power that lies behind their feelings.

When you're stuck in a rut, it's easy to get caught up on how you need the perfect doctor.

Lessons like Emma and Clara's prove that a physician or health advisor is only a part of the solution.

The biggest change comes from the smallest adjustment you make for yourself.

ANTHONY: Thank you so much, Dr. Katy, for sharing your story and the stories of your patients with our readers.

Please tell us a little about your practice and how our readers can get in touch with you if they have any questions.

DR. KATY MORTER: Morter Wellness Center is an alternative family health clinic in Bentonville, Arkansas.

Using gentle mind-body approaches, Drs. Ted and Katy Morter help clients overcome subconscious neurological and physical patterns that prevent them from living their BEST life.

Email: drkaty@morterwellness.com

Phone: 479-268-4477

Website: morterwellness.com

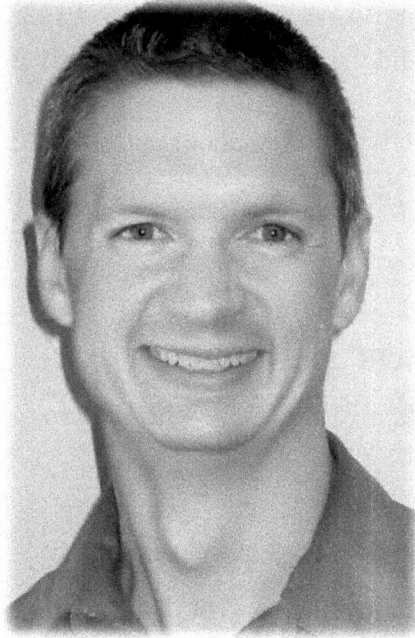

DR. KEVIN MORFORD

*Shares Inspiring Stories of Relief from
High Blood Pressure, Diabetes, Obesity and Tremors*

VOLUME ONE

ANTHONY: Welcome Dr. Morford. Please tell us about your patient, Eric, and his inspiring wellness journey.

DR. KEVIN MORFORD: Eric was a man who had just turned 60. While his life was great filled with family and success, he suffered from a myriad of health problems: High blood pressure, borderline diabetes, eighty pounds overweight, and developing an uncontrollable tremor in his hands.

Years spent behind a desk, eating whatever was available, trudging through the day, and just getting by had taken its toll.

Like most people, a plethora of health issues and weight gain sort of snuck up on Eric. Sure he noticed his body changing and those extra pounds starting to show up.

But he mainly attributed them to his age and genetics. Maybe most importantly, it was hard for him to see how his lifestyle really fit into the puzzle and was clueless when it came to improving it.

That's what made this story so interesting to me. Without really knowing how or why he wanted the changes, Eric sought help for himself.

He wasn't miserably unhappy. But he also wasn't experiencing joy and freedom at the levels he desired. Instead of having a pre-determined specific goal, he wanted to simply feel better, feel like himself, and feel alive again.

The first time I worked with Eric I was afraid I caused a heart attack. We were doing a workout together where I was showing him how to begin exercising again.

After just ten minutes, he had to excuse himself to the restroom and I wondered if he'd come back. We'd done a set of exercises for the chest and upon coming up off the bench following his third set of this move Eric got dizzy, light-headed, and frightened.

I remember even making a mental note of where the heart defibrillator was in the vicinity. Eric hadn't worked out in years, maybe decades, and was pushing himself to follow his old routine.

Those initial moments of worry and caution flipped a switch for Eric though, it was a flashing warning sign stuck right in his face that something needed to change.

It was really amazing at how willing he was to change the way he ate, add exercise into his daily routine, and get chiropractic adjustments when he needed them.

In one month he lost ten pounds, had more energy, suffered from fewer aches and pains, and his sessions at the gym were moving from those initially brutal ten minutes to lasting an hour. He felt good and you could see it in everything he did!

But that's not the greatest part of the story.

What impressed me most about Eric was how he made these changes a transformation. It wasn't a quick fix, get what you want and go back to the old ways thing. He completely refigured his mindset about who he was and what he was capable of achieving.

The sense of accomplishment and the energy and freedom he felt in himself motivated further action and inspired others. His lifestyle became one dedicated to feeling the highest levels of vitality and joy. The results inevitably followed.

After one year Eric had lost almost seventy pounds. He was taken off of almost all his medications and those he still needed were drastically reduced in dosage.

He became more active working in the yard and started running 5K events proudly sharing his times and experiences. The excitement he felt was palpable when he shared stories of having to go shopping for new clothes significantly smaller to fit his new, lean physique. And Eric glowed when other people remarked how great he looked.

My favorite story was one he shared after a trip to the doctor's office. While having his pulse and blood pressure checked by the nurses they made a comment on how healthy his values were.

They made a quick comment that based on Eric's pulse being so healthy they assumed he must be a runner. The smile on his face was ear to ear as he relayed telling those nurses, "I am now!"

Months prior he would have never imagined trained healthcare professionals complimenting his health. That day and those nurses confirmed his effort and dedication bringing a whole new level to his satisfaction.

People ask Eric how he did it. They assume he must have had some procedure, found a magic bullet, and some even worried he had fallen ill.

But the truth is, Eric used simple practices to achieve great results.

He ate more fruits and vegetables, dedicated himself to exercising, got adjusted as his body needed, drank plenty of water, and avoided doing the things we all know we shouldn't do in the first place.

It was even astonishing for him how simple the answers were. Dessert went from cake to bowls of fruit. Sipping on soda became sipping on water.

Exercise shifted from dread to anticipation. He even found he liked vegetables! This was all it took for a true transformation that affected every area of his life.

Five years later, Eric hasn't lost a beat. That transformation was indeed permanent. He is healthier at 65 then he was at 55, maybe even 45.

The renewed vigor has moved him into finding new hobbies, accepting different challenges, and finding fresh adventures.

Today Eric freely plays with his grandkids, goes on dream vacations, and lives each day with a fresh new perspective on how wonderful we can feel and how truly great life can be.

ANTHONY: Okay Dr. Morford, you have me motivated now... time to start eating better!

Who do we have up next?

DR. KEVIN MORFORD: This is the story of a woman who came to my office hoping to find relief for low back pain and inspired me instead.

Jenny was a wonderful woman to be around. Friendly, funny, polite, and she managed to put a smile on your face by just being in the room.

Talking with her on the phone before she ever entered my office, I never imagined I was speaking to someone confined to a wheelchair and carrying a diagnosis of a rare neurological disorder I had never heard of before.

It was only her warning right before our phone conversation ended that allowed me the time to look up the extremely uncommon condition.

Talking with Jenny showed how strong she was. Having first noticed symptoms at the age of 18 with foot drop, visits to neurologists became a norm over the next 30 years of her life.

During this time the condition progressively worsened with no cure known and the continual progressive decay a daunting reality.

Her condition was genetic, at least as far as they could tell. Years of doctor's visits considered every possible scenario for conditions including Parkinson's disease, Strokes, Multiple Sclerosis and Lou Gehrig's Disease (ALS). MRI scans, blood tests, CT imaging, and more became a normal part of Jenny's life.

When finally discovering the true diagnosis, it provided only temporary relief. With no options for a cure and a slow decline inevitable, even the doctor's told her they needed to see her only once a year. And that visit was to simply find out how far the disease had progressed.

It took only the most glancing observation to see how her disease was affecting her.

Besides the wheelchair, she required glasses that got continually thicker and had special lenses designed to keep the muscles of the eye engaged amidst fatigue.

Dexterity of her fingers was waning and her balance, even in moving from her wheelchair to her bed, was deteriorating at a rate that scared her spouse who wondered what would happen if he were out of the house and Jenny fell.

I wondered silently to myself how long could this possibly go on. Facing this reality was daunting to say the least.

But that never stopped Jenny. She worked out every day pulling herself out of her wheelchair and doing whatever exercises her failing hands would allow. She was open to new exercises that engaged her mind and stimulated her nervous system. Despite a disease that might make someone wonder why they should bother, Jenny took care of her body eating healthy foods, getting chiropractic adjustments, and doing whatever she could to support her.

When some thought she should stop, unsure of the need to struggle for a life of disappointment and heart ache, she saw living as the reason to keep going.

Where so many others would have quit long before, Jenny honored something deep within herself that called her to experience the beauty of life that maybe someone in her position is uniquely capable of fully understanding.

This story doesn't have a miraculous happy ending. Jenny's neurological disorder continues its slow debilitating deterioration of her body. I can say proudly that I helped her in that I at least eliminated her back pain, and in a time frame that I had thought nearly impossible.

This at least allowed her to work out with more energy and greater zeal while bringing back a bit of her zest for life.

What makes this story so amazing though, is how Jenny showed me that even in the worst of circumstances, there is something we can do.

Even when life seems determined to put us down, our heart and our love for living can build us back up. She's never quit despite all the questions on why she should bother to continue. She's honored herself in everything she's done for 30 years taking care of her body and appreciating the subtle nuances of life most take for granted.

Mark Twain said, "Courage is not the lack of fear. It is acting in spite of it." Jenny showed me what true courage looks like and her inspiration lives on in everyone who's heard her story.

ANTHONY: What seems to be the underlying theme in people who have had such success?

DR. KEVIN MORFORD: I've really seen two differences that stand out to me when I look at how some people have been able to experience great success in their health.

First, they become dedicated to themselves. It may have an extrinsic goal, like doing it for family, but their reason for sticking with it and finally reaching that goal was only done with a deep compassion and love for themselves.

If you don't value you, it's very hard to continue doing something positive for yourself.

The second difference I see is that those who find success often keep it very simple. They make a simple plan that will be easy to follow and stick with it.

I see people struggle constantly with complicated diets or drawn out programs. But those who make real change, real transformation, do so by keeping things simple.

ANTHONY: Thank you so much, Dr. Morford, for sharing your story and the stories of your patients with our readers.

Please tell us a little about your practice and how our readers can get in touch with you if they have any questions.

DR. KEVIN MORFORD: Based in Edmond, Oklahoma, we are a company dedicated to not only delivering the highest quality healthcare, but to educating our clients on how to experience the highest levels of health and freedom through their own actions.

We do this by showing people simple, easily applied tools for daily living so that they activate their body's natural ability to heal and fully realize the vibrancy and vitality within their bodies.

In doing this, clients become empowered to take charge of their health and their lives feeling the energy and freedom that comes with a healthy, vibrant body.

Phone: 405-844-4492

Website: chiropractic-now.com

createsimplehealth.com

Social: facebook.com/ChiropracticNow

facebook.com/DrAprilMorford

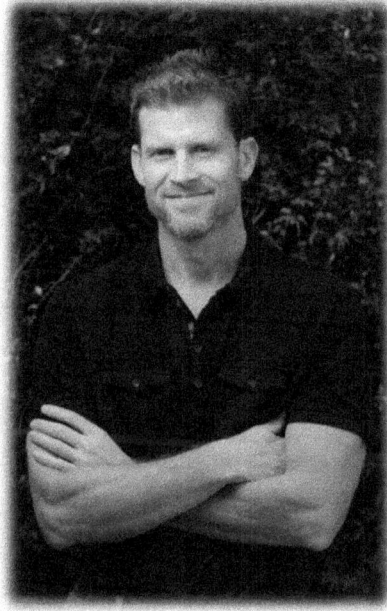

DR. MATTHEW BUCKLEY

Shares Inspiring Stories of Relief from Migraines, Fatigue, Fainting, Incontinence, Anxiety, Depression, Low Libido and Lyme Disease

ANTHONY: Welcome to the Wellness Journeys interview series, Dr. Buckley.

Please tell us about your personal wellness journey.

DR. MATTHEW BUCKLEY: Like many alternative practitioners, I was driven into the field of natural and energetic medicine due to my own health challenges.

As a teenager growing up in the Midwest I was active with athletics, but started to experience fatigue without any explanation. This fatigue gradually worsened through my undergraduate work at Illinois State, and began to accompany aches and pains that made me envision what 95 years old was like at the age of 21.

Like anyone else, I explained my dilemma to several medical doctors, and was eventually directed through the HMO process of seeing a psychiatrist for depression.

While I was certainly depressed, much of my depression was stemming from the fact that I was ill and nobody seemed to have any idea what was wrong with me. The standard blood tests and urinalysis revealed nothing.

After trying paxil and Zoloft for a couple months, my intuition led me to give up on those drugs as they were clearly not solving my problems.

Upon graduating from Illinois State, I took a job working as an engineer at John Deere and struggled to make it through the days. I could literally sleep 10 hours and feel like I needed another 5.

At no point in time was I ever out of shape. It was quite the opposite. I was working out frequently thinking that I just wasn't in good enough shape. I had no idea about the function of adrenal glands and how I was rapidly depleting them, impairing an already weak immune system.

After about a year at John Deere, I found myself having a conversation with a friend of a friend attending Chiropractic College, and became intrigued at the thought of getting the body to heal itself and figuring out what was wrong with me.

That conversation was a pivotal point in my life, as I doubt I would be alive today if I continued the path I was on then. Shortly thereafter, I enrolled at Logan College of Chiropractic. While attending Chiropractic College I encountered many chiropractic techniques, learning the chiropractic view of health.

I discovered that virtually every natural form of health care, including Traditional Chinese Medicine (TCM), homeopathy, Ayurveda, and naturopathy looked at health from a vitalistic viewpoint.

Vitalism looks at the whole individual with regard to all health problems, not focusing simply on symptoms and their treatment. In essence vitalism looks for the cause and how various body components and systems work in harmony to maintain homeostasis or body function.

This made sense to me. Likewise, techniques known as Applied Kinesiology and Chiro + Plus Kinesiology very much embraced other aspects of health, in comparison to a straight structural approach, as does much of chiropractic.

I was actually dealing with a significant toxic body burden, complicated by chronic infections including Epstein Barr Virus (EBV), parasites, candida, and Borrellia (Lyme disease), complicated by adrenal exhaustion.

As I began looking into the genetic picture of my problem, I found that my genetic profile was actually very similar to many who are dealing with Autism.

In short, genetic mutations (MTHFR, GSTP1) set me up for being a relatively poor producer of the body's most important detoxifying chemical, glutathione, which ultimately led to the seemingly complex neuro immuno endocrine disorder that I was dealing with.

ANTHONY: Thank you, Dr. Buckley, for sharing your personal success story with our readers. Please tell us about your patient, A.C.

DR. MATTHEW BUCKLEY: In July of 2013, A.C. came to see me with complaints of:

1) Brain fog/inability to concentrate, think, read, find words, and memory loss

2) Auditory hallucinations

3) Painful stomach cramping with alternating diarrhea and constipation her entire life

4) Chronic fatigue, with occasional black outs and fainting spells

5) Locking, sore, stiff joints, shooting pains and sore muscles.

6) Skin problems - hives, eczema, itchiness

7) Migraines

8) Urinary incontinence

9) Vomiting mucus in the morning

10) High anxiety with a history of abusing anxiety medication.

AC was 25 when she came in to see me, having found me through a referral.

She had described a childhood filled with sickness, along with multiple doctors and doctor visits only to be told that her problems were fundamentally mental.

Among the issues she had brought up to her doctors, but was casually dismissed by all but one, was the possibility that she may have parasites. Her most recent MD entertained that idea and ran a blood test to screen for toxoplasomosis antibodies, which came back negative.

No other parasite testing was done. Needless to say, she was frustrated, depressed, and feeling very little hope when she came into my office.

I utilize a bioenergetic form of testing referred to as "Autonomic Response Testing" (ART) which is an invaluable tool for aiding in the diagnosis of many problems, especially chronic infections such as parasites. (I do not do stool testing for parasites due to the high rate of false negative findings in the world of stool testing.)

My examination of AC revealed that she was dealing with multiple infections, with tapeworm and toxoplasmosis being primary infections (in spite of the lab finding), and candida being a significant secondary infection.

When infections are present for an extended length of time, such infections break down the gut lining which then allows for undigested food to enter the blood stream and drive food sensitivities. AC was no exception to this, and was found to be sensitive to gluten and casein.

Additionally, ART also indicated AC to be suffering from pyroluria, a disorder which can decrease immune defenses, leading one to be more prone to parasites and other chronic infections while simultaneously causing severe neurotransmitter and hormonal imbalances.

AC was advised to adopt a paleo diet and given a combination of remedies to facilitate the elimination of the parasites and yeast, in addition to a combination of vitamins and minerals that were specific to AC's body based on ART testing.

I saw her monthly for ½ hour sessions to make adjustments to her program along with some applied kinesiology based body work.

Within one month, she stopped having the morning vomiting, was less constipated, had less abdominal pain, and her allergies seemed far less severe.

ART indicated that she was improving with her infections, but they were not clear, and wouldn't clear completely for at least 6 months.

After 1 year, her body and mind were functioning on a completely different level.

She was no longer dealing with debilitating fatigue, depression, and was brimming with confidence to go to school and pursue a career in natural health. In her last visit with me she thanked me for my guidance and said, "You saved my life."

ANTHONY: You truly are a life saver, Dr. Buckley! Do you have another inspiring patient success story for us?

DR. MATTHEW BUCKLEY: In May of 2014, BT came in to see me having the following complaints:

1) Brain fog

2) Abdominal bloating

3) Back pain

4) Depression

5) Anxiety

6) Poor libido

BT was a 31 year old male avid outdoorsman, with numerous long backpacking trips under his belt.

Additionally, he loved to play basketball, but for the past 6 months had noticed that his brain and body wasn't working like it used to.

Work stress was high, but his recent deterioration suggested that something else was going on.

I ran some blood work on BT which came back looking deceptively good. He did show for a low normal range of white blood cells, and a low normal CD 57 which is a general screen for lyme infections.

Antibodies for lyme were negative. All other markers were normal. Low white blood cell counts are suggestive of chronic infections.

ART indicated a very different picture than what the blood work depicted, and matched his symptomotology much better than the blood work did. The energetic testing indicated that BT was dealing with a variety of parasites, tapeworm, threadworm, and hookworm in addition to lyme.

BT was put on a paleo diet, along with remedies to address the parasites and lyme, along with bi-monthly office visits for body work. We combined those with daily home use of an inversion table to help decompress an injured L5 spinal disc.

Within 1 month, he reported that his brain fog was lifting and his energy was improving.

WELLNESS JOURNEYS

Within 2 months, everything had improved so much that he did a 3 day hike with his brother in Big Bend State Park.

It took 6 months for the infections to appear to be cleared from his body.

His brain and body were functioning like he expected them to be, and he felt like he had his life back on track. He continues his long hikes and has even resumed playing basketball.

54

ANTHONY: Those parasites sure are pesky, but they're no match for modern natural medicine.

Now tell us about your patient who had undergone radiation for a tumor on her brainstem and what you were able to do for her.

DR. MATTHEW BUCKLEY: In November 2005, GF, a 43 year old female, entered my office having recently undergone six weeks of radiation for a tumor on her brainstem. This was her second round of radiation.

Prior to that round of radiation, this same tumor had been "removed" surgically, and the area was treated with a series of sessions of radiation to control the tumor growth.

When she entered my office, her primary complaints were:

1) Fear of the regrowth of the tumor.

2) Weakness in her right leg, which began following the radiation.

3) Weakness on her entire left side of her body, with numbness on the left side of her face.

4) Low energy/brain fog

5) Poor appetite

6) Daily headaches

Upon examination, it was revealed that GF was dealing with a significant toxic body burden which was being exacerbated by chronic infections. Autonomic response testing indicated her mercury amalgam dental fillings and root canal were major stressors to her system.

My approach in managing GF's case at this point was to strengthen her body by supporting her detoxification systems (liver, lymph, kidney, and gut), her endocrine system, while simultaneously supporting a gentle approach to knock down the infectious and toxin burden.

I saw GF once a week for 3 months where I supported the nutritional and detoxification program I put her on with gentle chiropractic and applied kinesiology.

During that 3 month time frame I had her consult with a local biological dentist about performing a dental revision, which would involve removing her toxic mercury amalgam fillings along with her root canal.

At around the 3 month mark, and feeling stronger than she had in a while, GF went back to the dentist for him to actually do the work to clean up the problems in her mouth.

After this dental work, we modified her program to be more focused on mercury detoxification. I continued to see her twice a month after that for another 6 months, and then have seen her about once to twice a month since that time.

She has had follow up imaging from her oncologist which confirmed that the mass which had previously been prone to growing, had actually shrunk since her last visit with him.

She is now working again full time, with good energy, feeling and strength completely returned to her entire body, free of headaches and brain fog.

Her case is a great example of the need for a much-disciplinary approach to someone dealing with chronic illness.

ANTHONY: Thank you so much, Dr. Buckley, for sharing your encouraging patient stories with our readers.

Please tell us a little about your practice and how our readers can get in touch with you if they have any questions.

DR. MATTHEW BUCKLEY: Our Kinsei office is located in Austin, Texas. For over 12 years, we have served the people of Austin, and surrounding areas, with cutting edge holistic services for restoring and maintaining their youth.

From infants to elderly, non-toxic and non-invasive modalities have helped those in need when their bodies were breaking down, as well as keeping performance at a top level.

We have helped many people overcome Back/Neck/Disc Problems/Joint Pain, Chronic Fatigue, Adrenal/Thyroid Dysfunction, Allergies, Autoimmunity, Autism, ADHD, Chronic Infections, Diabetes, and Digestive Distress.

Through diet, customized nutritional programs, functional lab work (using optimal values as opposed to lab normals), and advanced diagnostic techniques, solutions to complex problems can be obtained.

Email: drbuckley@kinseimindbody.com

Phone: 512-327-1771

Website: kinseimindbody.com

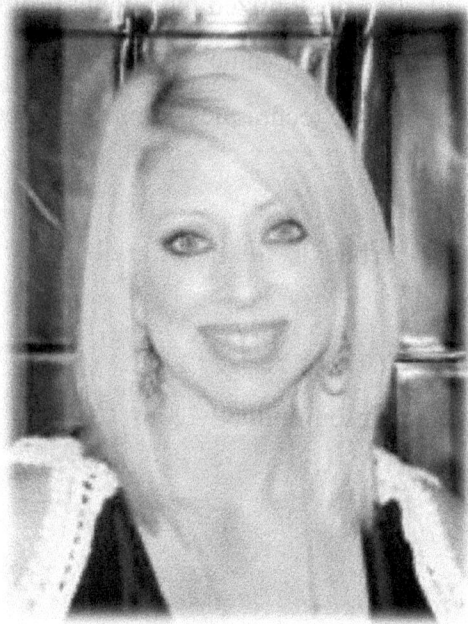

DR. ANGELA SONNIER

Shares Inspiring Stories of Relief from Ectopic Heartbeats, High Blood Pressure, Migraines, Degenerative Disc Disease and Arthritis

VOLUME ONE

ANTHONY: Welcome Dr. Sonnier. Please tell us about your personal wellness journey.

DR. ANGELA SONNIER: During my second pregnancy, I suffered from migraines and ectopic heartbeats which lead to high blood pressure and triggered migraines.

At the beginning of my second trimester, I was wearing a 24 hour heart monitor and ordered on bed rest. I was only one year into my chiropractic career and it abruptly stopped.

I was seeing a neurologist, cardiologist and a gynecologist monthly. I ended up in the ER for high blood pressure despite their pharmaceutical efforts.

At this point, I decided to see a chiropractor which helped keep the migraines at bay and through adjustments, trigger point therapy and acupressure, we were able to control my blood pressure.

I was told by my medical doctors I would be lucky to make it to full term and most likely would be facing surgery to correct the electrical misfires in my heart as soon as I had my son.

WELLNESS JOURNEYS

Despite their dire prognosis, I carried my son to 36 weeks (4 weeks longer than they predicted) and avoided surgery since "miraculously" my heart rate and rhythm returned to normal. I attribute my "miracle" to seeing my chiropractor regularly.

VOLUME ONE

ANTHONY: I'm glad to hear everything worked out well with you and your son!

Now tell us about your BioFreeze customer that became a patient and his inspiring wellness journey.

DR. ANGELA SONNIER: In my second year of practice, I noticed an elderly gentleman coming in often to purchase BioFreeze. I never had the chance to speak to him at the office since he came in during office hours while I was treating patients.

My CA informed me he said that I couldn't help him. I happen to see him at our local Heritage Festival and finally had the chance to ask him why he was using the biofreeze.

He said he was 81 years old and had both neck and back fusions and just used it to control his pain. He again stated I couldn't help him. I convinced him to come see me anyways.

He had an extensive history including degenerative disc disease in both cervcal and lumbar regions in addition to hyperkyphosis of the thoracic spine.

When I asked him what he misses the most about not being able to look up; he stated he just wanted to look at the moon with his wife again.

I used a chiropractic adjusting tool and active release technique along with PNF stretching to improve the joint motion above and below his fusion in his cervical spine.

Within a month of seeing me, he came into the office excited to tell me he had to move his rearview mirror up in his car! With continued care, he now is able to look at the moon. He has been a patient of mine for over 4 years now and always informs me when it's a full moon!

VOLUME ONE

ANTHONY: How nice that you were able to give him renewed health at age 81!

Please tell us about your young patient that suffered from severe headaches and how you were able to help her.

DR. ANGELA SONNIER: I have a four year old patient whose mother was referred to my office by another patient. She was nearly in tears telling me she has been to every doctor she could think of to help her daughter with the severe headaches she was experiencing.

She had no other medical problems and all the traditional medical test were normal. She was told her daughter was just wanting attention. She knew this was not true.

She told me how she was at the movies the previous Saturday and had to leave because her daughter was screaming out in pain.

Upon exmination, it was clearly evident she had cervical subluxations at c1/c2, c3/c4. I always like to have the parent feel the area where I find the subluxations before I adjust the child to educate them on what is causing the pain.

Post-adjustment, I have them feel the area again to ascertain the difference between whats normal alginment and what's not.

She came in once a week for one month and now comes in once every two months for her wellness adjusment. She went from having migraine headaches weekly to having only one "regular" headache since her treatment began.

I see her often at the elementary or local town events and she always runs up to give me a hug and yells "Still no bad headaches!"

VOLUME ONE

ANTHONY: Those hugs must be one of the greatest rewards of your job!

Next, please tell us about your patient who was unable to sleep in her own bed before seeing you.

DR. ANGELA SONNIER: I had 68 year old patient come into my office for lower back and hip pain. She had ankle surgery four months prior. She had to use a knee chair for four weeks, then wear a boot for another four weeks.

Once she started rehab she was suffering from hip and back pain. Her medical doctor had ordered physical therapy three times a week for six weeks.

When she entered my office, she was using a walker due to the hip and lower back pain and still had trouble with her ankle. She had so much pain she was unable to sleep in her bed; she was sleeping in a recliner.

Upon examination, she was suffering bilaterally from severe overpronation of her feet.

In addition to addressing her hip and lower back pain with spinal manipulation; I began working on correcting the overpronation of her feet using kinesiotaping and Myofascial release and PNF stretching.

She began seeing me three times per week and by her fourth visit she was telling me she was now sleeping in her bed most of the night. She continued seeing me three times per week for another month.

At the end of month two she was walking without her walker and able to sleep through the night in her bed.

She continues to see me once a month for her maintenance on her hip and lower back and we are now addressing an old shoulder injury that was surgically repaired but despite therapy she couldn't lift her arm out to the side without using her other arm to assist.

We've been working on it once a week using passive range of motion, kinesiotaping, and PNF exercises. She has gone from a 0/5 in motor function to a 2/5 in less than two months.

VOLUME ONE

ANTHONY: That is great progress in such a short period of time!

Got any more stories for us?

DR. ANGELA SONNIER: A short one… I have 75 year old patient with severe arthritis in both his hands and wrists.

Initially he was unable to open his palm all the way; his thumbs remained turned inward toward his palm.

He is a farmer and definitely uses his hands daily. Through Myofascial release technique of both his fingers and his wrists he is able to use his hands more with less pain.

He maintains motion and flexibility appointments every two weeks.

ANTHONY: Thank you so much, Dr. Sonnier, for sharing your story and the stories of your patients with our readers.

Please tell us a little about your practice and how our readers can get in touch with you if they have any questions.

DR. ANGELA SONNIER: At Vinton Chiropractic, in Vinton, LA, I focus on providing superior service combined with quality care.

All patients are thoroughly examined and complete medical history is obtained. Every patient has a unique response to chiropractic care. No two patients receive the exact same treatment plan.

I have over 7 years in chiropractic practice and focus on getting their pain level down as quickly and effectively as possible through spinal manipulation, Myofascial release, and kinesiotaping techniques.

VOLUME ONE

These are followed by educating my patients with at-home exercises to improve posture and therapeutic exercises to improve spinal joint motion and flexibility which increases the patient's overall wellness.

Educating patients on how the muscles interact with the joints leads to a better understanding of what normal function feels like whereby increasing the patient's awareness to abnormal body function.

My goal is to teach patients how to thrive in life instead of how to survive in life.

Email: drangelasonnier@yahoo.com

Phone: 337-409-0822

Social: facebook.com/VintonChiropractic

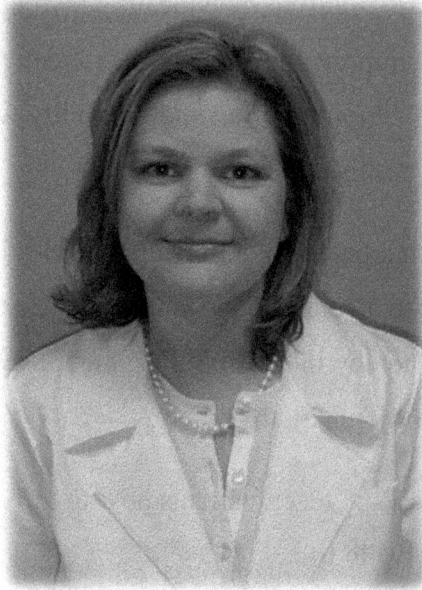

DR. CARISSA HAMILTON-TOUPS

Shares Inspiring Stories of Relief from
Lower Back Injuries, Muscular Knots and Migraines

VOLUME ONE

ANTHONY: Welcome Dr. Hamilton-Toups.

I hear there's an interesting wellness story behind how you decided what you wanted to be when you grew up.

DR. CARISSA HAMILTON-TOUPS: I went to a chiropractor my whole life. My grandfather would not go to a medical doctor, but would go to his chiropractor. So, those values were instilled in my mother.

Anytime, even at the age of 5, if I got a crick in my neck it was off to the chiropractor for instant relief.

When I was in high school I attended UL (formally USL) softball camp. It was a really intense camp. While sliding into second base my lower back began to hurt. I was staying in a dorm and was not allowed to bring my car with me. I could no longer run or bend over.

After painfully realizing that I could no longer deal with the pain I called my mom. We lived about 25 minutes from where I was staying. She left work and drove to the softball field to pick me up.

WELLNESS JOURNEYS

I remember limping to the car and having trouble getting in the passenger seat.

Mom asked me if I wanted to get my things and go home. I was so disappointed that I would have to give up the rest of the camp. I thought about it for a minute and said, "No, would you mind driving me back home to get an adjustment from the chiropractor?" She didn't hesitate to say, "Of course".

We made the trip back to my hometown of Crowley to see my chiropractor. My chiropractor watched me walk into the treatment room and immediately asked me, "What did you do?" It was that obvious!

After one treatment I got up off of the table feeling like the pain that I just felt was a distant memory. It was gone. Instant relief!! Mom drove me back to camp and I completed the rest of the activities with no problems.

If there was ever an instance in my life where I knew what I wanted to be "when I grew up" it was that moment. To be able to provide people with natural healthcare pain relief is amazing!!

VOLUME ONE

ANTHONY: Instant pain relief, it's the best kind! Thanks for sharing that story.

Next, I believe you have a patient success story for us.

DR. CARISSA HAMILTON-TOUPS: One day our office gets a call from a gentleman who was a police officer out of town. Let's call him Harry. Harry wanted to come in because of some shoulder blade pain.

Once he arrived, during examination, I found a huge swollen muscular knot located to the left of the edge of his shoulder blade. Upon discussion, he said that this had been going on over a week. He was in so much pain that he had his adult son dig his elbow into the swollen muscle in the back while Harry lay on a counter.

They were trying to release the muscle. He had a portable TENS unit at his home and had tried using that on the muscle. Nothing that he did helped. He wasn't even sure what had caused this to happen.

After a thorough examination of the area I could tell that his Rhomboid muscles and Levator Scapula muscles were inflamed and swollen. I then suggested he try this new technique called Dry Needling that I had just taken a course in a few weeks prior.

The course was intense and took two separate full weekends to complete. I explained to Harry that I would be using small gauge needles to try and release the swollen muscle in his shoulder blade. The technique is designed to help the brain send a signal to the muscle to begin the healing process. Poor Harry was up for anything.

First I used my industrial TENS unit on the area. This machine contracts the muscles in the back over and over again to try and get them to release. He was of course reluctant because he had used his TENS at home with no relief. But, this helps the muscle relax a little so that I can Dry Needle the area better.

I then had him lay on my table and proceeded to "needle" the inflamed area. Normally, I would just go in a muscle once or twice with a needle, but this was a special circumstance. I "needled" the area probably five times trying to create as many small lesions in the muscle that I could to stimulate healing in that area. He said the procedure was completely painless. Harry barely felt a thing.

After treating that area I gave him an adjustment. He was already feeling relief but the knot was still present and would certainly take some time to go down. Harry seemed pleased and said he would be back the next day for another treatment.

The next day Harry entered my office with a grin from ear to ear. He showed his back to me and in amazement the swelling was COMPLETELY GONE! He said it was like it had never happened. He had been in pain for days upon days and in one treatment he was 100% better! I can't tell you how happy I was to hear this.

As a practitioner, we mainly see people that are hurting and miserable. I want to take their pain away as badly as they want to get rid of it. To see someone so happy that I was able to help him get out of pain quickly was such a humbling experience.

Harry is my best advocate. He has referred numerous people to my office for my services. We are constantly sending him Thank You cards for his referrals. I am so glad that I had the chance to treat him.

VOLUME ONE

ANTHONY: Painless needles are my favorite! Thanks again for sharing that story.

Next, I believe you have a bulging disc story for us.

DR. CARISSA HAMILTON-TOUPS: After years of losing patients to expensive traction therapy at large chiropractic facility in another town, I was able to find a traction table that was a fraction of the cost for my office. We were so excited to have this table and the results that could be obtained from it.

A patient came in one day, let's call him Mike. Mike had lower back pain and would let it go till he was in horrible pain and could barely walk. He was a tall heavy man with a family history of back issues.

The pain would go down his left leg and make it difficult for him to move around. After an examination and history of Mike I told him we really needed to do an MRI. He agreed and had the study done immediately.

The results showed that he had a large 10 mm left paracentral disc extrusion at L4/5. In other words he had a huge disc bulge in his back.

Mike and I discussed treatment options. He was adamant that he didn't want surgery. I told him that his only other option that I could determine was trying a treatment plan of traction on his lumbar spine. He agreed and so the treatment plan commenced.

He came in religiously for treatment. We would use the traction table on every visit and pull him for about 15 minutes. After approximately two to three months he was completely out of pain.

And of course, when out of pain, out of mind. He stopped coming in for treatments and we didn't see him again for about two years.

Mike comes back into the office with lower back pain. If I remember correctly, he had lifted on something heavy that he should not have and caused this new episode.

VOLUME ONE

He repeated over and over again how he should have come in once a month for traction on his back to maintain all that he had accomplished but life got in the way. After examining him again I was troubled that the original 10mm disc bulge had possibly gotten worse. We ordered another MRI.

To my utter astonishment the original L4/5 10mm disc bulge was completely gone!! I called the facility that did the MRI and asked them if they could check it again against the original MRI.

Both of these studies were done at the same facility. The radiologist called me back and said that he was utterly amazed that the bulge completely retracted and wanted to know what we had done to cause it. Then after speaking to the radiologist I was told that the original bulge was actually 13mm not 10mm. WOW!!

When I relayed the information to the patient he was extremely pleased. We went back to our original treatment plan of traction of the lumbar spine.

ANTHONY: I think my back could use some traction table time. That sounds really good!

Do you have one more for us?

DR. CARISSA HAMILTON-TOUPS: One day, out of the blue, a man walked into my office. Let's call him Wilson. He had a horrible migraine headache. Wilson said that he had been to the chiropractor before, many years ago, and really needed an adjustment.

You could see the agony in his face. He agreed to be examined and X-Rayed because we had never seen him at the office before. I remember moving as quickly as I could, thinking how I would feel in his shoes.

While he was in the waiting room, painstakingly filling out his paperwork, some patients walked in with kids. Our floors were linoleum so everything in the office echoed and every noise was enhanced. The clamor was about to cause him to pass out.

VOLUME ONE

We had to move him into a dark room so that he could sit peacefully and complete his papers. Poor Wilson was about to vomit from the pain -- a common side effect of migraines. I had to keep a trash can near him just in case.

After taking films of his neck it showed that he had some rotation in his C1 vertebra. The skull sits on the C1 vertebrae and sometimes will cause a headache if rotated. This poor vertebra has the whole weight of the head on it, so it is understandable that it could cause a migraine if rotated.

I explained to Wilson that I needed to palpate the area and see if there could be a problem there. Sure enough I could feel that there was definitely a problem.

I administered a C1 adjustment to his neck in the seated position. Wilson felt immediate relief. The migraine was completely gone and the nausea as well. The relief was instant. He was so grateful for the relief. I have to say it was a great feeling to see him smile.

WELLNESS JOURNEYS

ANTHONY: Thank you so much, Dr. Hamilton-Toups, for sharing your story and the stories of your patients with our readers.

Please tell us a little about your practice and how our readers can get in touch with you if they have any questions.

DR. CARISSA HAMILTON-TOUPS: I have a solo Chiropractic Clinic located in Crowley, Louisiana. We offer a variety of services that best suites our patients.

The office employs a Massage Therapist and has done so for the past 4 years. We offer Dry Needling, Traction, Therapy, and Chiropractic services.

Phone: 337-783-3334

Website: crowleychiro.com

VOLUME ONE

Acknowledgments

WELLNESS JOURNEYS

I'd like to thank, once again, the wellness professionals that invested their valuable time into this project.

Drs. Katy and Ted Morter, IV

Dr. Kevin Morford

Dr. Matthew Buckley

Dr. Angela Sonnier

Dr. Carissa Hamilton-Toups

If you are a wellness professional and would like to become a contributor to a future volume of Wellness Journeys, visit RPMpublish.com and send me a note using the form on the Contact Us page.

Thanks,

Anthony Curtis

Wellness Professionals Directory

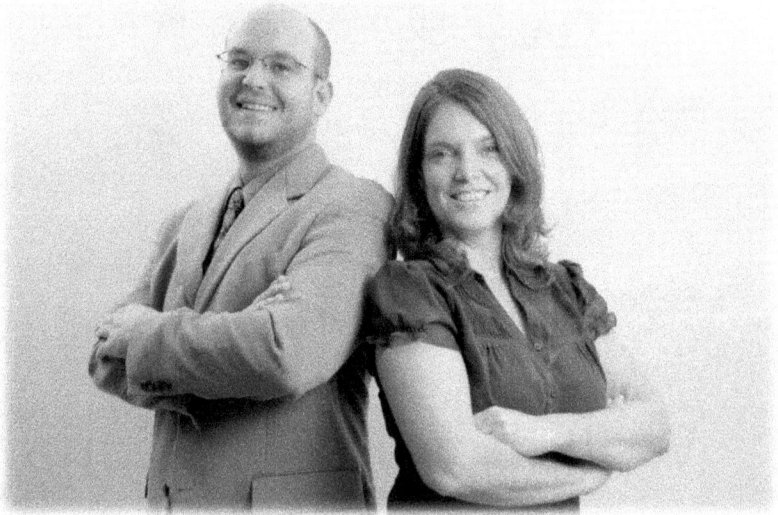

Drs. Katy and Ted Morter, IV – Bentonville, AR

Email: drkaty@morterwellness.com

Phone: 479-268-4477

Website: morterwellness.com

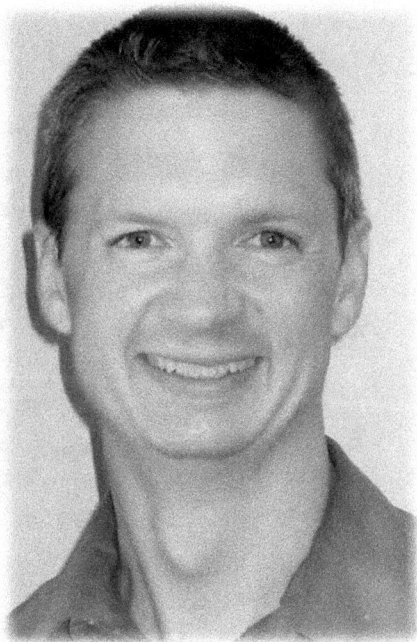

Dr. Kevin Morford – Edmond, OK

Phone: 405-844-4492

Website: chiropractic-now.com

          createsimplehealth.com

Social: facebook.com/ChiropracticNow

          facebook.com/DrAprilMorford

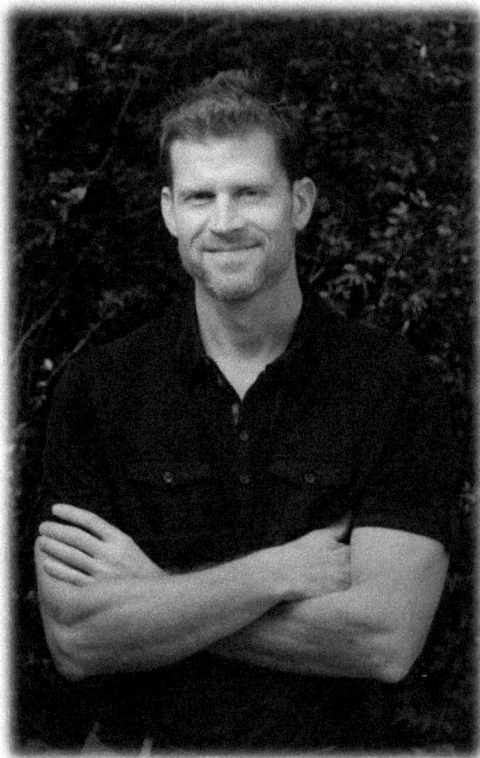

Dr. Matthew Buckley – Austin, TX

Email: drbuckley@kinseimindbody.com

Phone: 512-327-1771

Website: kinseimindbody.com

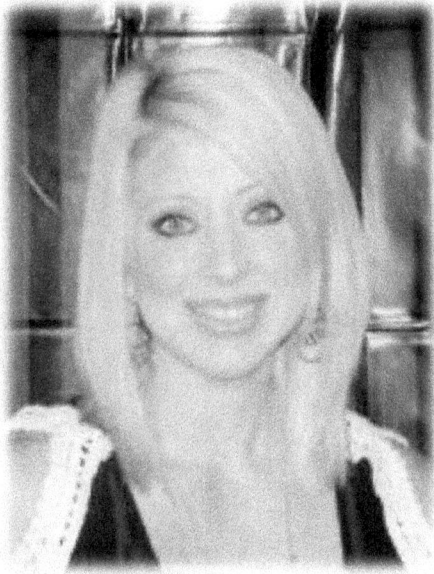

Dr. Angela Sonnier – Vinton, LA

Email: drangelasonnier@yahoo.com

Phone: 337-409-0822

Social: facebook.com/VintonChiropractic

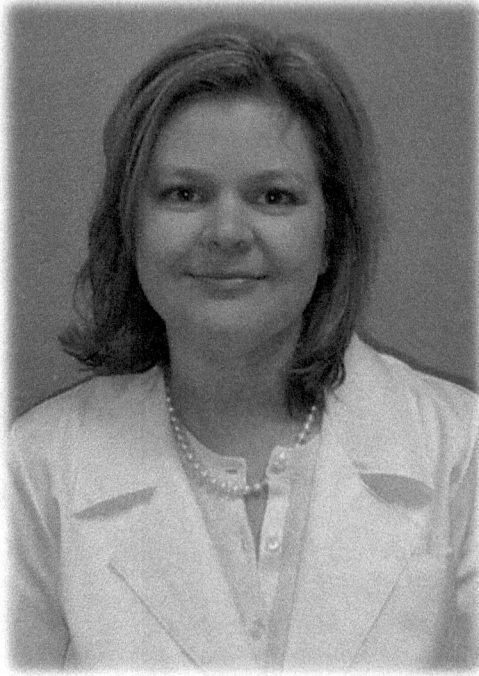

Dr. Carissa Hamilton-Toups – Crowley, LA

Phone: 337-783-3334

Website: crowleychiro.com